MW01114218

ALCOHOL/DRUG- DEPENDENT WOMEN

New Insights into Their Special Problems, Treatment, Recovery

Sheila B. Blume, M.D.

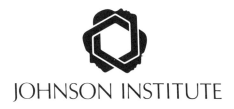

JOHNSON INSTITUTE

To the millions of women trapped by alcohol/drugs, and to those who have devoted their lives and careers to helping them.

Printed in the United States of America.

ISBN 0-935908-45-5

INTRODUCTION

We humans differ in many ways from our fellow creatures. Perhaps our most important anatomical feature is the human brain, which has made it possible for us to reshape the world around us. Yet that same brain has sought not only to change the way the world *is*, but also, by altering its own feelings, mood, and perceptions of reality, to change the way it *seems*. Throughout history and in all parts of the world, techniques have been developed to alter internal reality. Some have involved religious rites, meditation, sensory deprivation, fasting or dance, but most have achieved altered brain function through the use of a psychoactive drug. Societies in which mind-altering drugs have been readily accessible have often developed drug-related problems, particularly with those drugs capable of producing dependence. Alcohol has historically been the most important drug of abuse in Western society, and it remains so today, with nicotine perhaps a close second. However, the use of other sedative drugs and of marijuana, opiates, hallucinogens, and stimulants such as amphetamines or cocaine has also created significant problems, often in combination with alcohol abuse.

The alcohol/drug problem is one of the greatest facing contemporary society. In our eagerness to tackle it, though, there's always the danger of generalizing too hastily, of assuming that all alcohol/drug users are about the same and that therefore our ways of identifying, diagnosing, and treating their problems should be about the same. This booklet hopes to dispel that

---

Editor's Note: The term "alcohol/drugs" is employed in this booklet to emphasize that alcohol *is* a drug—just like tranquilizers, cocaine, marijuana, heroin, or any other mind-altering substance. Too often people talk about "alcohol *or* drugs" or "alcohol *and* drugs" as if alcohol were not itself a drug. We also sometimes use the term "chemical dependence" because it covers dependence on *all* these mind-altering substances and because it's short and simple.

myth as it explores our latest knowledge about the special problems of women in regard to alcohol/drugs.

For now, let's mention just two examples of how women's problems are special.

One problem is that in nearly all human societies, norms for what is or isn't permissible in regard to alcohol/drug use are different for men and women. In the early days of ancient Rome, to cite an extreme example, the law of Romulus forbade women to use alcohol, and some women were put to death by stoning or by starvation for violating that law. Although sex-related differences in drinking rules may sometimes protect women, they can also be destructive. It's interesting, for example, that the Roman law that forbade drinking by women also forbade them to commit adultery. Writers of the time explained that alcohol was forbidden to women because it made them sexually promiscuous. This same double standard of drinking and this same stereotype of the female drinker (or other drug user) as a lewd woman survive in American culture today. And they still provide a basis for the special stigma attached to alcohol/drug-dependent women. This stigma creates a barrier to identifying and treating these women, for it encourages individual, family, and societal denial and encourages the alcohol/drug-dependent female to remain in hiding.

A second example of women's problems in regard to alcohol/drugs relates to their special role as mothers. Recent research has shown that dependent mothers subject their fetus to risks of damage, including fetal alcohol syndrome and prenatal sedative and opiate dependence. In addition, alcohol/drugs may interfere with normal pregnancy and birth, causing such complications as premature or pathological labor. Moreover, alcohol/drug dependence often distorts early nurturing and mother-infant bonding. A special problem for the modern woman is the responsibility of being a single parent. When she suffers from alcohol/drug dependence, her children are likely to lack a stable caring adult. And so the damage done by these diseases passes from generation to generation.

4

Yet for all their difficulties, alcohol/drug-dependent women can and do recover. They and their families can be helped if they can be reached and treated. This booklet addresses itself to that important task by summarizing recently acquired knowledge about alcohol/drug problems in women and how to identify, diagnose, and treat them.

WOMEN'S USE OF ALCOHOL/DRUGS

Use Patterns

An important source of information about drinking problems is the general population survey. Such studies of drinking behavior in the general population have uniformly found that women drink less than men, are more likely to abstain, and have fewer drinking-related problems. Estimates of the relative prevalence of female and male alcohol problems have varied widely over time and according to the population studied. However, there's little doubt that drinking and alcoholism in women have increased considerably since the end of World War II. Moreover, during the past ten years clinicians have reported a remarkable increase in the number of alcoholic women, particularly younger women, appearing for treatment. The National Institute on Alcohol Abuse and Alcoholism estimates that in 1985 nearly 6 million American adult women were either alcohol abusers (nearly 2.5 million) or alcoholics (more than 3.3 million). This represents about 6% of the adult female population. By comparison, just over 12.1 million men, or about 14% of the male adult population, have serious alcohol problems. The proportion, then, is about two males to one female. To put it another way, about one third of all adults with drinking problems are women. Clinical experience with adolescent alcoholics yields a similar ratio.

Another source of information about the onset and prevalence of alcoholism over the years is the study of families of patients in treatment for alcoholism. Recent studies of this kind comparing 1983 data to 1969 findings have documented both an increased prevalence and an earlier onset of alcoholism in women over that 14-year period. So we have good reasons to be concerned.

Much of our understanding of the drinking patterns and problems of women comes from a comprehensive nationwide survey conducted by Dr. Sharon Wilsnack and her colleagues at the University of North Dakota. This project collected detailed information from over 900 women drinkers (sampled so as to include 500 "heavier" drinkers) and nearly 400 drinking men. The highest rates of both men's and women's alcohol-related problems (such as driving under the influence, belligerence, or interpersonal conflict), as well as the highest rates of alcohol-dependence symptoms (such as memory lapses or morning drinking), occurred in the youngest age group (21 to 34) included in the study. In men, the highest rate of heavier drinking was found in the same age group. Among women, on the other hand, the highest proportion of heavier drinkers was found in the 34- to 49-year-old group. This curious dissociation of heavy and problem drinking awaits further research.

However, the difference between male and female patterns is relevant to prevention and early intervention. In American men the heaviest drinking occurs in young adulthood, so men who maintain a pattern of heavy drinking or who increase their drinking into their late 30s and 40s are atypical and therefore merit special diagnostic attention. Among women, however, the rate of heavier drinking continues to climb (although not to levels as high as it does in males) beyond early adulthood and into middle life. Since women may begin their alcohol dependence at any age, and on the average do so later than men, prevention efforts must continue throughout a woman's life cycle. Programs that teach women how to cope with life problems without their relying on alcohol or other drugs are important components of prevention. But such programs shouldn't be limited to teenagers and young women; they should focus on women undergoing important transitions at any point in their lives. Examples would be prevention components in programs for battered women, displaced homemakers, and women going through divorce.

The Wilsnack study also found that the characteristics of women showing the highest rates of alcohol problems varied according to age. Risk factors for those in the youngest group surveyed (21-34) were being single (never married), childless, and not employed full-time. These were young women who had not assumed expected adult roles. Among the women aged 35-49, the highest problem rates were found among those divorced or separated, unemployed, or having children who did not live with them. These women had assumed but lost at least some of the adult roles. The oldest women in the study, aged 50-64, showed most alcohol problems among those who were married, not employed outside the home, and those having children no longer living with them—traits reminiscent of the so-called "empty nest" syndrome. This important study clarifies the relationship of alcohol problems to changing roles and transitions in women's lives, as well as to age.

Patterns of other drug use and drug problems in women have also varied during recent American history. Women have been the primary abusers of therapeutic drugs (both prescribed and over-the-counter). In the late nineteenth and early twentieth centuries, before legal accessibility to many drugs was severely limited by law, narcotic dependence was common in American women. Women of all social classes became dependent on a variety of "tonic wines" and medicinals containing opiates and purchased at the local pharmacy. One popular tonic, Vin Mariani, contained cocaine (as did Coca Cola) before the Harrison Narcotics Act of 1914. When such drugs became very difficult to obtain, women didn't shift in great numbers to illegal drugs. Instead, they became dependent on other prescribed drugs, such as the barbiturates and meprobamate of a few decades ago, and the amphetamines and benzodiazepines (minor tranquilizers) of today.

Today, American women remain more frequent users of prescribed drugs and less-frequent users of cigarettes, marijuana, cocaine, and other illegal drugs than men are. Although women begin alcohol/drug use at a later age than men and use them less frequently, differences in use patterns are less marked among young people today than in previous generations. Researchers have referred to the "vanishing difference" between the sexes in the use of alcohol/drugs by adolescents. Among teens, cigarette smoking has become as common among girls as boys. In addition, data from a 1985 national household survey by the National Institute of Drug Abuse indicate that among women of childbearing age (18-34), 30% reported having used an illicit drug at least once during the previous year, and 18% had done so during the previous month. So we must be seriously concerned about women's abuse of both illegal and prescribed drugs. Illegal drug use isn't just a male problem.

Hereditary Patterns

Some of the most important research in recent years has explored genetic factors in one's predisposition to alcohol problems. Family studies over many years have clearly demonstrated that alcoholism is far more common in the relatives of alcoholics than in the general public. However, special techniques are necessary to distinguish inherited from environmental influences. One such technique is the study of twins; another is the study of adoptees. Early studies comparing identical and fraternal twins involved only male subjects. As for adoptees, later research from Denmark showed a probable genetic influence for men but was inconclusive for women. However, the Stockholm adoption study, which involved 1,775 adults adopted by non-relatives early in life, has yielded much information on heredity patterns of alcohol problems in women as well as in men. By comparing records of alcohol-related problems in the offspring of biological parents with and without records of alcohol abuse, researchers were able to distinguish two patterns of heredity relevant to women.

The more common type of inheritance, called type 1, was seen in both sexes. This type was characterized by adult onset and less severe alcohol abuse (as measured by health and arrest records). Alcohol abuse by either biological father or mother, or both, increased the risk for alcohol problems by a factor of 3 in these adoptees. Environmental as well as genetic factors were important determinants of alcohol abuse in later life.

In addition, the researchers identified a less common, male-only pattern, type 2. It involved severe, early-onset alcohol abuse associated with criminality in both biological father and son, and revealed stronger hereditary influence than type 1. Neither the biological mothers nor the daughters of these fathers had an increased incidence of alcohol problems, but the daughters had a high incidence of multiple physical illnesses.

At our present state of knowledge it's fair to conclude that a genetic influence is probable in at least some alcoholics. However, the disease shouldn't be looked upon as hereditary—that is, present at birth and not preventable. The demonstration of environmental influences in these studies offers us clear opportunities for prevention, particularly in women.

Less is known about genetic influences on the origins of other drug dependences, but there also may be an increased risk of such problems in those offspring of alcoholic parents who have been adopted and raised by non-relatives—which indicates an inherited predisposition. A recent study by Cadoret and his colleagues offers evidence for this hypothesis. In that study, as in the studies on alcohol abuse, both hereditary and environmental factors proved to be important.

Physical Factors

Early studies of the male human body's reactions to alcohol assumed that the findings would apply to both sexes. Recent research has challenged this assumption.

Jones and Jones (referred to in the Greenblatt and Schuckit work mentioned in the bibliography) showed that women reach higher peak levels of alcohol in the blood than men, in response to a standard dose of absolute alcohol per pound of body weight. This is in part due to the higher proportion of water in men's bodies. Since alcohol consumed is dissolved in the total body water, a standard dose will be less diluted in a woman. The Joneses also found that, unlike males, their female subjects showed a great deal of day-to-day variability in peak blood-alcohol levels, correlated in part with the phases of the menstrual cycle, with the highest peaks occurring in the premenstrual phase. In practical terms, then, a woman will react more strongly than a man to an equivalent amount of alcohol and will likely be less able than a man to predict accurately the effect on her of a given amount of alcohol consumed.

Differences between men and women have also been found in their vulnerability to some of the late-stage physical complications of alcoholism. Compared to men, alcoholic women have been found to develop fatty liver and hepatic cirrhosis, as well as hypertension, anemia, malnutrition, and gastrointestinal hemorrhage, at lower levels of alcohol intake (even correcting for differences in body weight) for fewer years.

Although much has been written about changes in emotions and behavior during the menstrual cycle, few investigators have looked at women's drinking patterns in relation to those changes. In one study, nonalcoholic women reported that significantly more negative moods, more drinking to relieve tension or depression, and more solitary drinking had occurred during menstruation. Since these drinking patterns are characteristic of alcohol dependence, the menstrual cycle may influence the early development of pathological drinking patterns in women. Some women suffering from alcoholism have reported that their drinking tended to be heaviest just before their menstrual periods. Others have reported that they were introduced to the use of alcohol to relieve distress when they were given alcoholic beverages during their teens as a folk-medicine remedy for menstrual cramps. This use of alcohol, like other supposedly medicinal uses, should be strongly discouraged.

Very little is known about the effects of alcohol consumption on women's sexual functioning. Heavy drinking has been linked to infertility, lack of sexual interest, inability to reach orgasm, and a wide variety of obstetrical, gynecological, and sexual dysfunctions. An interesting set of experiments looked at changes in the sexual arousal responses of men and women to single doses of alcohol. In men, both self-reported feelings and physiological measurements of arousal increased in response to sexual stimuli when the subject believed he had consumed alcohol (whether or not he had actually received it). In women, however, there was dissonance between subjective feelings of arousal and physiological responses. Women who thought they had received an alcoholic beverage said they felt more arousal, whether or not they had actually consumed alcohol. However, actual alcohol consumption depressed physical arousal, even if the women *thought* they were more stimulated.

In a further study on orgasm in women, it was demonstrated that increasing levels of blood alcohol interfered progressively with the rapidity and intensity of orgasm. In spite of these negative physiological effects, studies of alcoholic women show that they often expect greater desire and enjoyment of sex when drinking (while at the same time they report a high incidence of sexual and reproductive dysfunction). This seeming paradox is probably due to the women's culturally-determined expectations that alcohol increases sexual desire ("Candy is dandy; liquor is quicker"). This is an important observation for clinical practice that may well apply to other psychoactive drugs as well. The expectation of a drug's effects and its actual physical effects often differ. A chemically dependent woman, faced with the necessity of abstinence from alcohol/drugs as a condition for her recovery, is likely to assume that she will have to sacrifice sexual pleasure in the process. Simple education about the deleterious effects of alcohol/drugs on sexual excitation and orgasm will reassure her that a satisfactory loving relationship is likely to yield far more sexual pleasure during her sobriety than was possible during her time of alcohol/drug abuse.

Alcohol/Drugs and Pregnancy

The Fetal Alcohol Syndrome (FAS) and other alcohol-related birth defects are a special problem of concern to women. FAS probably occurs in between one and two cases per 1,000 live births. Along with Down's syndrome and spina bifida, it's one of the three most frequent causes of birth defects associated with mental retardation. Of these three, it's the only one that is completely preventable. However, adequate prevention requires that obstetrical personnel identify women problem drinkers early in their pregnancy or, preferably, *before* pregnancy. Public education about the danger of alcohol to the fetus and the recommendation that pregnant women avoid drinking aren't sufficient prevention for women who are already alcohol/drug dependent. And when these women do become pregnant, they need treatment in order to become alcohol/drug-free, both *during* the pregnancy and *afterward*. Resuming alcohol/drug use after the baby is born will cause relapse, which will both interfere with adequate parenting and reestablish the other symptoms of the disease.

In addition to the fully-expressed fetal alcohol syndrome, drinking during pregnancy can result in a wide variety of other problems for the fetus, ranging from miscarriage to low birth weight and birth defects. The defects, called fetal alcohol effects (FAE) or alcohol-related birth defects (ARBD), are far more common than FAS. While FAS is usually seen in the offspring of alcoholic women who drink heavily during pregnancy, FAE can be observed in women with lower intakes of alcoholic beverages—intakes compatible with social or non-problem drinking.

Thus it's important to educate all women of childbearing age who may be pregnant or planning pregnancy. Both U.S. and Swedish studies of women who drank heavily early in pregnancy but were helped to stop alcohol use by the end of the second trimester (sixth month) have shown that it's possible to improve greatly the chance for a healthy baby. None of the infants whose mothers managed to stop drinking produced an infant with the full FAS. Infants of those mothers were also less likely to show low birth weight, neonatal distress, or birth defects. Likewise, experiments on animals have shown that the developing fetus can compensate for alcohol-related damage to some degree if alcohol intake is stopped during pregnancy. (Lyn Weiner has reviewed this evidence in the 1987 paper cited in this booklet's bibliography.)

The message this research sends to clinicians is clear. Even if a woman is already in early pregnancy and drinking heavily, she shouldn't be made to feel it's too late to help her current pregnancy. She should be strongly encouraged to enter treatment immediately; clinicians can keep her in treatment by taking advantage of her desire to produce a healthy baby.

There are no absolutely reliable estimates of the probability that an alcoholic woman who drinks during pregnancy will produce an infant with FAS or FAE. One study found a probability of 40%. However, a variety of factors including diet, the use of other drugs, prenatal medical care, physical health, number of previous pregnancies, and length and severity of alcoholism all seem to play a role along with alcohol intake. One retrospective study compared the children of 36 upper-middle-class and upper-class alcoholic women with the children of 48 alcoholic women who were on public assistance. The women differed significantly in race, marital status, parental alcoholism, and beverage of choice but not in alcohol intake. The women of lower socioeconomic status, who were Black (70%) or Hispanic (30%) and more likely to drink beer, contrasted with the White upper-class women, who preferred hard liquor or wine. The differences in the incidence of FAS and FAE were striking, with overt effects present at birth in 71% of the children of the public-assistance mothers and in only 4.6% of the children of upper-class mothers. However, even though these children of upper socioeconomic-class mothers were considered normal at birth, their birth weight was lower, and 21% later showed signs of attention-deficit disorder. (Details may be found in the paper by Bingol and colleagues, cited in the bibliography.)

Opiates haven't been shown to cause birth defects similar to FAS. However, women physically dependent on opiates at the time of delivery do put their infants at risk for neonatal withdrawal syndrome. They also increase the risk of stillbirth and complicated labor. Such pregnant women and newborns require intensive and specialized medical care in order to avoid or minimize complications and distress.

Stimulants such as amphetamines and cocaine have been reported to cause miscarriage, premature labor, and other obstetric complications. Infants of mothers who have used these drugs may be jittery and irritable at first, and later depressed. Marijuana use has been suspected as a contributor to birth defects and may act in conjunction with other factors such as alcohol and malnutrition. Cigarette smoking has been associated with decreased birth weight and prematurity.

Sedative drugs, including sleeping pills and tranquilizers, can also present significant problems for pregnant women. Use of Diazepam (Valium) early in pregnancy has been implicated in birth defects in animals, as have barbiturates. All sedatives, if used in large doses up until delivery, can produce infant drowsiness and poor feeding, followed by a neonatal withdrawal syndrome that will cause continuing distress and will interfere with mother-infant bonding.

Alcohol/drug use during nursing should also be avoided, since alcohol and some other drugs enter the breast milk. The folk-medicine practice of giving alcoholic beverages to nursing mothers to "help the milk" has no basis in scientific fact and should be discouraged.

With the increased frequency of teenage pregnancy in our society, prevention of adolescent alcohol/drug use (including tobacco) takes on a special urgency. The treatment of a chemically dependent pregnant woman should be considered a medical emergency and given the highest priority. Fortunately, the wish to protect the health of her unborn child is a powerful motivator for treatment in many pregnant women.

Psychological Factors

There's still a great deal of uncertainty about possible psychological factors that may predispose some people to alcohol/drug dependence. Studies of clinical populations fail to distinguish factors that might have been present before the onset of illness from those that are products or concomitants of the disease itself. These distinctions can only be made in studies employing a longitudinal design—research that follows subjects from childhood or adolescence into adulthood to discover which early traits predict later alcohol problems. Few longitudinal studies of alcohol/drug problems have included female subjects. Mary Cover Jones, in a long-term follow-up study (see bibliography), identified general feelings of low self-esteem and inability to cope as predisposing factors in preteen and teenage girls who later became problem drinkers. This contrasted with the predisposing factors in males, which were aggressiveness and rebelliousness. Unfortunately, the number of problem drinkers in Ms. Jones's study was small.

Fillmore, in a 27-year follow-up of drinking among American college students (see bibliography), found that factors predicting problem drinking in later life differed considerably between males and females. The best predictor of later problems for women was a high score on the "feeling adjustment" scale, composed of such items as drinking to relieve shyness, drinking to get high, drinking to be "happy," and drinking to get along better on dates. Among men, those with mild rather than serious alcohol-related problems in college were most likely to show up in the problem-drinker group at follow-up. Although these studies don't establish the existence of an "alcoholic" or "addictive" personality, they do tend to confirm the clinical observation that women often begin their alcohol/drug dependence during periods of emotional distress, using the psychoactive substance as a medication.

One psychological theory that has focused specifically on the alcoholic woman has been that of sex-role conflict. The theory is based on socially accepted definitions (actually stereotypes) of masculine and feminine behavior. It postulates that women who develop alcoholism have strong identification with feminine roles at the conscious level but strong *unconscious* feelings of masculinity. This disparity creates a conflict at least partially relieved by alcohol, which has been found to enhance feelings of femininity in both normal and alcoholic women.

The concept of sex-role conflict has been further developed to include women with conflict between conscious masculine strivings and unconscious feminine identification. A study by Beckman (see bibliography) at the University of California investigated conscious and unconscious masculinity and femininity in 120 female alcoholics, 119 non-alcoholic women, and 118 women in treatment for psychiatric and emotional problems. The author concluded that although a sex-role conflict between "unconscious masculinity" and "conscious femininity" was more prevalent among alcoholic women than among the normal controls, less than one quarter of the total alcoholic sample showed this pattern of conflict. When sex-role conflict was defined to include both conscious femininity and unconscious masculinity and the reverse, there was no significant difference between the alcoholic women and the controls in regard to the incidence of that conflict. Sixty-six percent of the alcoholic women, 72% of the treatment controls, and 71% of the normal controls scored feminine on both conscious and unconscious measures. Those alcoholic women who manifested sex-role conflict differed from the other alcoholic women in showing lower self-esteem and a higher incidence of having had an absent parent during childhood. Identification of alcoholic women suffering from such conflict is certainly an important consideration for treatment, but sex-role conflict cannot "explain" alcoholism.

Social Factors

Whatever the genetic and psychological predisposition of any individual woman, to develop chemical dependence a woman must be exposed to alcohol/drugs in a context in which she finds it personally acceptable to use the substance. Thus social and cultural norms and values that influence access to various drugs, and attitudes toward their use, play an important part in the development of chemical dependence. The socialization of women that makes it more acceptable for them to visit physicians, to acknowledge and seek help for physical and emotional symptoms, and to use prescription psychoactive medicines helps shape patterns of female alcohol/drug dependence. Studies of medical practice have also shown that physicians prescribe psychoactive drugs more readily to women than to men for the same complaints. On the other hand, it has been more socially permissible (or even expected) for males to use illegal drugs. And women dependent on such illegal drugs as heroin and cocaine often report that they were introduced to the frequent or heavy use of such drugs by husbands or boyfriends.

Social values and customs are critically important in both causing and preventing alcohol/drug problems. Educational prevention programs attempt to decrease the acceptability of high-risk drinking and of alcohol/drug use by minors. However, attractive advertising campaigns in the electronic and print media that glamorize the use of alcoholic beverages remain a major source of influence on the public. In recent years this advertising has increasingly been aimed at women, who, it has been claimed, may be targeted by the beverage industry as a "growth market." After all, the "average" American woman drinks only half as much as her male counterpart. Ads showing glamorous models in fashionable attire, or women in unconventional settings, seek to associate drinking with success, excitement, and being a "liberated woman." Tobacco advertising has done likewise. "You've come a long way, baby" is the marketing slogan of a cigarette designed for women.

As was previously mentioned, the alcohol/drug-use patterns of adolescents have shown progressively fewer male/female differences in recent years. Since females attain higher blood-alcohol levels than males in response to equal doses of alcohol, and since women and girls tend to be lighter in weight, any change in social norms that expects a woman to "drink like a man" (or requires males and females to consume any other drug at the same dosage level) will be especially damaging for women. Prevention programs should stress these differences.

Another important social factor affecting use patterns is the stigma attached to women who use alcohol/drugs. Although it may be argued that this stigma discourages alcohol/drug abuse, it produces a great many pernicious consequences, particularly for the chemically dependent woman.

As was mentioned in the introduction, even as far back as ancient Rome, Western society has associated sexual availability or promiscuity with women who drink. This idea persists in twentieth-century America as part of the triple stigma borne by alcoholic women. First, they carry the same general stigma as male alcoholics. Although many Americans accept the disease concept of alcoholism, this acceptance is still very superficial. When asked directly, the same people who agree that alcoholism is a disease also feel that it's a disease that happens to weak and/or immoral people and that it's "self-inflicted."

Secondly, women in Western society are expected to adhere to a higher moral standard than men, at least in theory, and are therefore more despised when they fail to live up to expectations. This increases the stigma attached to alcohol/drug dependent women.

Finally, the assumption that women who use alcohol/drugs are sexually promiscuous is particularly damaging. This assumption hasn't been confirmed by research. Wilsnack and her associates (see bibliography) investigated this question as part of the large national survey of American women mentioned above. The women were asked if they had ever had the experience of being less particular about their choice of a sexual partner when they had been drinking. Only 8% of them reported such an experience, and although fewer (4%) among the lightest drinkers answered yes, the moderate and heavier drinkers (11% and 12%) didn't differ. Such results do little to support the idea that drinking makes women "loose." On the contrary, the evidence shows that this societal stigma has promoted sexual victimization of women by considering women who drink as acceptable targets for male aggression.

The Wilsnack study also asked if the women subjects had ever had the experience that someone who had been drinking became sexually aggressive toward them. Sixty percent of all women, in approximately equal proportions of light, moderate, and heavy drinkers, responded yes. Similarly, a study by Fillmore (see bibliography) on social victims of drinking found that women who drink in bars (that is, who were exposed to others while drinking) were far more likely to be victimized, even if they were not themselves heavy or problem drinkers.

On the other hand, problem drinkers or those who often drink heavily were most victimized, among both men and women.

Recent direct evidence of this sexual stigma (that women drinkers are sexually promiscuous) has been found by Dr. William George and colleagues (see bibliography), who studied the reactions of college students to a videotape of a young adult date scene. Both male and female students rated the woman in the scene more sexually available and more likely to have intercourse if the scene showed her ordering an alcoholic beverage rather than a soft drink. Furthermore, she was rated even more likely to be available if the male paid for the drinks than if they split the cost.

In light of the above, it's not surprising that many alcoholic women who reach treatment have histories of being the victims of rape and other abuse. And clinical experience with women in treatment for other drug dependence has been similar.

Finally, this social stigma also acts as a major barrier to the identification and treatment of the women who desperately need help. Since the alcoholic woman grows up in the same society as the rest of us, she applies this stigma to herself and keeps her problem hidden because of guilt and shame. She tends to drink alone, often in her kitchen or bedroom, and the nature and extent of her drinking or other drug use is often not appreciated by her family and friends until she has reached an advanced state of her disease. In addition, although she may seek help repeatedly from medical facilities because of her failing health, nervousness, and insomnia, the stereotype of the alcohol/drug-addicted female as the "fallen woman" makes health professionals less likely to suspect these diagnoses in their well-dressed, socially competent female patients. The chemically dependent woman seldom recognizes the basic nature of her own problem, since to *her* the alcohol/drugs are not her problem. Rather, they are her attempt at solving the many other problems she perceives as troubling her. It's no surprise, then, that she often leaves the doctor's office with a prescription for additional sedative drugs rather than with a referral for addiction treatment.

CLINICAL ASPECTS OF ALCOHOL/DRUG PROBLEMS IN WOMEN

Course and Symptoms of the Disease

Most researchers agree that women coming to treatment for alcoholism differ from their male counterparts in a number of ways. Women start drinking and begin their pattern of alcohol abuse at later ages but appear for treatment at about the same age as male alcoholics. This points to a more rapid development or "telescoping" of the course of the disease in women. Alcoholic women are more likely than men to be divorced when they enter treatment or to be married to or living with an alcoholic "significant other." They're more likely than the alcoholic man to relate the onset of pathological drinking to a particularly stressful event. Women are more likely to have histories both of suicide attempts and of previous psychiatric treatment. Their motives for entering treatment and the problems they perceive as relating to alcohol are more likely to be health and family problems, whereas for the male, job problems and trouble with the law, particularly arrests for driving while intoxicated, are more prevalent.

Women alcoholics have a high incidence of obstetric and gynecological difficulties, and they develop cirrhosis more rapidly than males. Various studies have shown that women more often have histories of other drug dependence along with their alcoholism—particularly dependence on tranquilizers, sedatives, and amphetamines. Female alcoholics are also more likely to have such symptoms of psychological distress as anxiety and depression and to have lower self-esteem than their male counterparts. Some of the same characteristics have been reported for opiate-dependent women, particularly the psychological symptoms, low self-esteem, and the "telescoped" course of the illness.

Diagnosis

In diagnosing alcoholism in a woman, the volume of alcohol consumption is an important consideration. It's well established that alcoholic women, on the average, drink less than men (as much as 45% less, in one study) but experience the same degree of impairment. It's particularly important to recognize that use of other sedatives may contribute to the woman alcoholic's impairment. Instead of a morning drink, she may have a morning Valium; her nightcap may contain less alcohol and more sedative drug. Thus alcoholism shouldn't be diagnosed as a function of the *quantity* of intake alone. Drinking and other drug-use patterns, and changes in personality and functioning, are the primary considerations.

Diagnostic criteria for the various psychoactive drug dependences are the same for men and women. Screening methods such as the "CAGE" questions or the Michigan Alcohol Screening Test (MAST) have been utilized for both sexes. However, a diagnostic questionnaire specifically for women was developed by Dr. Marcia Russell at the New York State Research Institute on Alcoholism for the State's FAS prevention campaign. This diagnostic questionnaire (Appendix 1) and instructions for using it (Appendix 2) can be found at the back of this booklet. Also included is a modified version adapted to test for both alcohol and other drug problems (Appendices 3 and 4).

Laboratory testing may also be helpful. A recent report on 100 alcoholic women referred for their first episode of treatment in Stockholm, Sweden, found that two standard blood tests—mean corpuscular volume (MCV), which measures the volume of the red blood cell, and gamma glutamyl transferase (GGT), a liver enzyme—were of diagnostic value. Although neither test is specific for alcoholism, two-thirds of the patients tested higher than normal in one or both of them.

Subtypes of Alcoholism

There have been many attempts to develop systems for subtyping patients suffering from alcoholism. The most useful of these subtypings, particularly for women, is the distinction between primary and secondary alcoholism. Secondary alcoholism is defined as alcoholism associated either with preexisting diagnosable psychopathological states or with such states developing during a prolonged period of abstinence. Primary alcoholism arises without such a history.

Most alcoholic patients appearing for treatment are of the primary type. Among men the most common secondary alcoholism is that associated with sociopathy. In women the most common type is so-called "affective alcoholism," that is, alcoholism secondary to depression. This latter pattern may be seen in one-fifth to one-quarter of a typical female treatment population. Diagnosis must be based on a careful life history, since the presence of depressive symptoms at the time of treatment won't differentiate between primary alcoholism with secondary depression and primary depression with secondary alcoholism. Once a woman is diagnosed as a secondary alcoholic suffering from affective alcoholism, an appropriate long-term treatment plan would include continuing contact during sobriety, with attention to possible recurrence of depression. Early treatment of such recurrence can help the patient maintain her sobriety and well-being.

The same principles apply to the treatment of women with other drug dependences that are secondary. Less often than with depression, there's a clear history of a primary anxiety disorder, such as panic disorder or agoraphobia, in an alcohol/drug dependent woman. It's essential that the treatment plan for such a patient be tailored to her individual need. Alcohol/drug dependence has also been found to be associated with a variety of eating disorders in women, including anorexia nervosa, purging bulimia, and compulsive overeating. These eating disorders may precede or accompany the alcohol/drug disorder. In many of the complex so-called "dual diagnosis" cases of chemical dependence and other psychiatric disorder, the anxiety or depressive disorder is secondary to the dependence. Although both disorders may require specific treatment, relapse of a secondary psychiatric disorder is less probable once the patient has recovered from the chemical dependence.

Casefinding

Although our best estimate of the ratio of males to females suffering from alcoholism in the United States today is about 2 to 1, our best current national statistics reveal a male-to-female ratio in alcoholism *treatment* closer to 4 to 1. So it seems likely that women are seriously underrepresented in treatment; or, to put it another way, the alcoholic woman remains hidden. One possible explanation is that the three most effective early intervention programs available today, drinking-driver rehabilitation, public-intoxicant intervention, and employee-assistance programs, have one characteristic in common: they reach a far greater proportion of male problem drinkers than females. Since the problems that motivate women to go into treatment are most likely to be health and family problems, primary casefinders for the female will be physicians, other health professionals, social and family service agencies, and attorneys.

Alcoholic women often visit their physicians. A recent study of two gynecological practices conducted by Dr. Andrea Halliday and her associates (see bibliography) found that 12% of the 147 patients who came in for periodic gynecological care qualified for a diagnosis of alcohol abuse or dependence. Of 95 women who sought treatment for premenstrual syndrome (PMS), 21% satisfied these diagnostic criteria for alcoholism. The average woman of this group was in her thirties (childbearing age). The average education was beyond high school. These women were in many ways typical of middle-class women in outpatient medical care.

An additional report in the *Journal of the American Medical Association* in January of 1988 found that 17% of a group of women attending a university hospital medical clinic for the first time scored in the alcoholic range on the Michigan Alcohol Screening Test. In the same study, 26% of male patients were found to be alcoholics. This male-to-female ratio of 1.5 to 1 surprised the authors. The study illustrates once more that a good place to find alcoholic women is in the doctor's office.

TREATMENT CONSIDERATIONS

Early Treatment

It's important to remember during the detoxification phase of treatment that women are frequently dependent upon other drugs in addition to alcohol. A careful, complete history should be taken from family members as well as from the patient if possible. The woman entering treatment for alcoholism may continue to deny the extent of her prescribed drug use or may purposely under-report such use in the hope that she will still be able to rely on her favorite prescription drug "if she really needs it," even after she has given up drinking. The clinician should be alert for delayed withdrawal symptoms such as tremors or seizures, insomnia, anorexia, hallucinations, or delirium. These may be due to withdrawal from benzodiazepines or other sedatives that have a longer duration of action than alcohol.

A complete physical examination is important because of the alcoholic woman's vulnerability to physical complications. Women of childbearing age should of course be tested for pregnancy.

Psychiatric evaluation should include not only present diagnosis but a differentiation of primary and secondary disorders, as was discussed above. A sexual and reproductive history with attention to both problems and expectations will aid in treatment.

In the post-detoxification phase of treatment, family involvement is critical. Each child of an alcoholic mother should be evaluated for fetal alcohol effects if there is a history of drinking during pregnancy. Even if no such damage is evident, the children need help in understanding the effects of their parent's disease on their families, and in understanding and expressing their own needs and feelings. Likewise, spouses and other close family members or friends can profit from education, counseling, and self-help groups.

Especially if the alcohol/drug-dependent woman is a single parent, the absence of reliable child care can make it impossible for her to enter an inpatient program or to concentrate on her treatment if she has already entered one. Anxiety about her children's well-being may be a formidable barrier to treatment. At present there are only a few women's treatment facilities that are able to house both mother and children. Help with child care may be the critical factor in reaching chemically dependent women.

Early-recovery problems for a woman may include depressed mood, intense feelings of shame and anxiety, and low self-esteem. All-female therapy groups and/or separate programming for women have been recommended by some clinicians. While there's no clear research evidence for the superiority of either single-sex or mixed-sex treatment, either can be successful if the clinical staff is aware of the special needs of women. This awareness includes sensitivity to the effects of societal stigma, to the socialization of women, and to the practical economic problems faced by women in employment, housing, and credit.

For example, women in our society are typically socialized to place the needs of others (especially of family members) before their own, as part of the role of nurturer. They're discouraged from directly expressing their own needs and feelings (especially their anger). These women may unconsciously expect others to sense their needs and fulfill them without their having to ask, as they strive to do for others. The ideal wife/mother, in this way of thinking, is the one who arrives with a cold glass of juice just before her husband/children/parents realize they're thirsty. When others fail to recognize a woman's unspoken wishes, she may feel resentful, hurt, or worthless. In attempting to establish a functional alcohol/drug-free life, such a patient will profit from learning to evaluate realistically her own needs in relation to those of others and to express herself directly.

Self-esteem issues are closely related to the values of society. Stigma has already been discussed. However, other aspects of identity are also important—for example, occupation ("I am what I do"). In contemporary American society, "women's work" has much lower status than work usually associated with the male. Although increasing numbers of women are part of the work force, women are still concentrated in low-prestige jobs and in 1987 earned an average of only 70% of what men did (and this figure represents a rise from the 62.5% reported for 1979). Work performed in the home is assigned essentially no social or economic value. ("Does your wife work?" "No, she's a housewife.") When employees perform home tasks, they're usually paid at minimum wage. Furthermore, the vast majority of working women who are also married continue to carry the responsibility for all or almost all of the cleaning, laundry, cooking, shopping, and child care.

In short, women are often underpaid, underemployed, under-valued, and overstressed. Striving for perfection in these competing areas of life will produce problems in any woman. But in a recovering chemically dependent woman who is attempting to allay feelings of guilt and shame and to make up for lost time, the problems will be even more intense.

In addition, a woman's identity is often defined through her relationships to others. She is somebody's daughter or some-body's wife, and at marriage she gives up her name (really her father's name) for her husband's. She may even be identified through a former relationship—for example, as so-and-so's ex-wife or widow. Building self-esteem may well require attention to these issues.

Minority-group membership may intensify women's social, economic, and self-esteem problems. The therapist needs to understand and appreciate the norms and values of the subculture to which the patient belongs so that intervention and treatment planning will be culturally appropriate. For example, a mixed-sex therapy group may be a poor choice for a patient whose culture doesn't permit men and women to discuss personal matters together. A woman from such a culture will do better in individual treatment with a female therapist or in a woman's group. Hence it's of little value to recommend that a woman attend an evening AA group at which both sexes are present if her subculture frowns on such activity. On the other hand, the therapist can take advantage of a subculture's strong extended family system to help the patient develop social supports.

Several reports have suggested a high prevalence of alcohol/drug problems among lesbian women. The special problems of this group shouldn't be ignored or belittled in treatment on the grounds that "alcoholism is alcoholism, and it's all the same." Attention must also be paid to the issues of physical and sexual abuse and incest, which have been found more common in the histories of women in treatment for alcohol/drug dependences than in non-addicted women.

Contact with other recovering alcohol/drug-dependent women should be encouraged, since they may serve as positive role models and assist with practical techniques in maintaining abstinence. Self-help groups, including Alcoholics Anonymous (AA), Narcotics Anonymous (NA), Cocaine Anonymous (CA), and Women for Sobriety (WFS), provide contact with recovering women. According to a recent survey by Alcoholics Anonymous, 34% of its members are now women.

Self-help groups serve many other important functions in early recovery. The societal stigma attached to alcohol/drug dependence, so troublesome in the outside world, is absent in the self-help subculture. On the contrary, the new member finds herself for the first time in a roomful of people who proudly identify themselves as alcoholics, cross-addicted alcoholics, or drug addicts. Their smiling self-label is met with a friendly greeting from the other members of the group. The highest status that can be achieved in the group is "recovering alcoholic" or "recovering addict." A woman can attain that identity by taking the first of the twelve steps (for AA, NA, or CA) and by allowing the group to help her remain "clean and sober, one day at a time."

Self-help group members offer much practical advice, built on years of group experience, on remaining abstinent. The new member will also be encouraged to choose a sponsor, who will give her close individual attention. Special beginners' meetings and "step" meetings are available in many places to help members understand and work the twelve-step program in their early months of abstinence. Most chemically dependent women have felt desperately alone in their battle against alcohol/drugs. Whatever friends are left to them are often drinking or using other drugs themselves. As was mentioned earlier, many of these women are divorced, separated, or living with active alcohol/drug abusers. Even supportive family members, baffled and hurt by their disease, have a great deal of difficulty understanding their experience in early recovery. The self-help group is a ready-made social network of understanding people. Although inpatient and outpatient therapy groups offer similar opportunities to break through isolation and learn to trust, these groups are by their nature temporary. But trust learned from peers in treatment groups, if extended to self-help, offers a lifelong supportive experience.

Women in treatment may also profit from reading about the lives of other women who have shared their experiences. In addition to the personal stories in the AA and NA "big book," autobiographies by women who have recovered may also be helpful in inspiring hope. (A number are listed in the bibliography.)

Finally, a few words should be added concerning the pregnant patient. She will require intense medical as well as psychological support. As was mentioned earlier, there are no precise estimates of the risk of birth defects in women who drink and/or use other drugs throughout pregnancy. However, longitudinal studies of pregnant women have shown that women who were able to achieve abstinence from alcohol before the third trimester didn't produce infants with the full fetal alcohol syndrome. Thus it's important to take advantage of the patient's concern for the health of her unborn child, if she continues the pregnancy. Patients shouldn't be made to feel that all the alcohol damage is inflicted early in pregnancy and that later treatment for alcoholism in the pregnant patient will be of no help to her child. However, it's also important that the treatment not be focused only on the pregnancy, with the goal of merely staying abstinent until delivery. A goal of full recovery from chemical dependence will be necessary for both the mother's health and for the adequate nurturance of her offspring.

Special techniques are needed to detoxify pregnant women addicted to opiates or sedatives. Those maintained on methadone may give birth to infants requiring medical detoxification, but there's no evidence that these infants are at risk for birth defects similar to those associated with FAS.

Continuing Treatment

Later on in recovery, after initial abstinence has been established, a wide variety of issues may arise in treatment, depending upon the individual psychological, interpersonal, social, vocational, and physical status of the patient and her family.

Affectional and sexual problems may have been put aside for future attention while concentration is focused on early abstinence. Later on in treatment a more thorough exploration of the woman's experiences, expectations, feelings, and present relationships may be indicated. Some studies have found that women in early recovery tend to avoid sexual relationships. This is often a useful strategy to prevent the kind of premature liaison that's looked upon as a magic way out of addiction. Before the chemically dependent woman has established her own sense of mastery and self-esteem, she will usually be unable to enter into a satisfying intimate relationship. However, she may also harbor the unrealistic fear that she won't be able to enjoy sexual relations without alcohol/drugs. This expectation may interfere with reestablishing a good sexual relationship with an appropriate partner (for example, her husband) or may cause her to avoid potential relationships when she's otherwise ready to undertake them.

Any woman who has taken drugs intravenously or has had sexual relations with partners who have used IV drugs should be offered confidential testing for the HIV virus that causes acquired immune deficiency syndrome (AIDS) and for hepatitis B carrier status. If she's found to be positive for either virus, she should receive expert counseling on her potential for infecting others (including a child, should she become pregnant). She should also receive support and counseling on the importance of abstinence in maximizing her chances of maintaining her present state of health, if HIV positive, and on the need for close medical follow-up. On the other hand, all women in treatment need education about high-risk sexual practices and about precautions that are likely to reduce the chance of HIV infection.

Other issues that arise after initial abstinence has been established include strong and conflicted feelings toward family members, particularly in women who are daughters of alcoholics and who grew up in dysfunctional families. There is growing literature based on clinical experience in treating adult children of alcoholic parents—for example, the book by Dr. Timmen Cermak listed in the bibliography. Adults brought up in these families often have exceptional difficulty in establishing trust, expressing their feelings, and forming intimate relationships. In addition, there's often an intense ambivalence toward the alcoholic parent. In accepting the diagnosis of her own chemical dependence, the recovering woman must face the distasteful fact that she has become like her parent, in just the way she vowed she would never do.

It's important, then, that she be given the opportunity to explore both the similarities and the differences between her own illness and behavior and that of her parent. This process will both allow her a deeper understanding of her parent and will help her establish her own identity. This will usually lead her, if she has children of her own, to reexamine the dynamics of her present family and her role as a mother.

The very last problem a recovering woman is often ready to admit is that she has been a less-than-perfect parent. Many women in early treatment cling to the notion that, with all their other failures, at least they were always good mothers. This denial begins to fall away, without any need for confrontation, when they've developed enough self-esteem and courage to want to communicate at a feeling level with their children and to hear about their children's experiences, resentments, hopes, and expectations. This kind of experience becomes possible at different times for different women, but it often takes many months to achieve. Treatment and self-help for family members should begin at the same time as the treatment of the patient, if not before, but additional joint sessions with both the patient and other family members may be helpful well into recovery if the desired communication hasn't been achieved.

Other problems that sometimes arise as treatment proceeds include dependence on a therapist, counselor, or other person—often a hostile dependence that may interfere with progress in individual counseling. One way to avoid this problem is to use group treatment from the beginning, supplemented with individual or family sessions when needed. If individual treatment is chosen, it's even more important for the therapist to insist on self-help involvement and to avoid taking responsibility for the patient's abstinence.

At times during treatment, anxiety or insomnia may be so severe as to threaten sobriety. Since the usual medicines used to treat these symptoms carry their own risk of dependence, deep relaxation techniques and other non-drug methods are preferred. The symptoms sometimes present an opportunity to help the patient reexamine the way she has structured her time, her commitments, and her activities. As a result, she may decide to change the way she lives so as to allow time for exercise, rest, and recreation.

Depressive symptoms present a different problem. When a depressed mood is clearly a reaction to life events, counseling alone may be sufficient to tide the recovering woman over a period of mild depression. In women whose history reveals primary depression with secondary chemical dependence, or whose depressive symptoms are severe and/or unrelated to life events, treatment with antidepressant drugs should be considered. In any case, continuing group and/or individual treatment will be required along with increased attendance at self-help groups until the depression is relieved. Evaluation of suicidal risk should be ongoing in any depressed chemically dependent woman, and hospitalization may at times be necessary.

Health issues that aren't resolved with the establishment of abstinence should be approached in continuing treatment. Women who are dependent on alcohol/drugs often have poor eating habits and may need help in understanding their nutritional needs. Gynecological problems and infertility may need attention. One health problem that should be raised by the therapist, if it's not raised by the patient, is smoking. Recovering women should be helped and encouraged to break their nicotine dependence. Having overcome their addiction to alcohol/drugs, they're prepared to understand what's needed to quit smoking. They may require a time-limited group program in addition to their ongoing treatment. Several of the self-help groups now have smoke-free meetings or nonsmoking sections. There's no simple formula for determining the best time during recovery to stop smoking; it's not unusual for a few attempts and relapses to precede the final success.

PROGNOSIS

There has been no systematic research on the relative effectiveness of various treatment programs designed for women. In general, male and female alcoholic patients with comparable demographic characteristics (marital status, employment, social stability, e.g.) and at comparable stages of illness do equally well in the same treatment settings. For example, the two-year outcome studies performed by the CATOR (Chemical Abuse/Addiction Treatment Outcome Registry) group, involving 1001 adults (about one-third female) treated in five Minnesota inpatient chemical dependence programs, showed little difference (see bibliography). Their one-year follow-up of over 1800 adolescents (about one-third female) showed girls significantly more likely to report total abstinence (50.3% versus 39% for boys). Girls who had been physically abused, had legal problems, had attempted suicide, or who were depressed when treated were less likely to report abstinence than others.

In contrast, two recent follow-up studies dealing with adult alcoholic women found that those with depressive disorders decreased their drinking more than others. In one of these studies, however, the depressed women continued to show more psychological symptoms than others a year after treatment, in spite of their decreased alcohol use. These and other studies indicate that there's no reason to believe that female patients are harder to treat than males or are less apt to recover.

Mortality rates are high for alcoholic women who don't achieve recovery. One study by Dr. Elizabeth Smith (see bibliography) followed 103 women treated for alcoholism at two hospitals in St. Louis. Eleven years after discharge, 31% of the women were dead, at an average age of 51.5 years. Their mortality was 4.5 times the normal rate, and they lost an average of 15 years from their expected life span. Those who attained abstinence, however, didn't show higher mortality rates.

PREVENTION CONSIDERATIONS

A useful way to conceptualize primary prevention is in terms borrowed from the model of infectious disease: agent, host, and environment. The agent in this model is the alcoholic beverage or other drug; the host is the woman (or girl) at risk, and the environment is the social and physical milieu in which she lives.

Measures that limit access to alcohol/drugs, such as minimum purchase age, control of alcohol and tobacco advertising, regulations that govern the prescription of psychoactive drugs, and control of illegal drug traffic, are aimed directly at the agent. Important measures specific to women involve education of health professionals to be cautious in prescribing sedatives, stimulants, and minor tranquilizers to women, particularly to those who may have an alcohol/drug problem. Warning labels on prescription and over-the-counter medicines that interact with alcohol/drugs may also aid prevention.

Measures aimed at the host include different forms of education about alcohol/drugs, and a variety of techniques to help women cope with stressful situations and transitions without relying on alcohol/drugs.

Health-warning labels are now required on cigarette packages and advertisements, but efforts to legislate similar labels on alcoholic beverages have as yet been unsuccessful. On the state and local level, however, laws requiring the display of warning posters wherever alcoholic beverages are sold have had more success. These posters often carry specific messages about the danger of birth defects. Such poster legislation was first passed in New York City in 1983. Since that time, the State of Georgia and many cities, including Los Angeles, Philadelphia, Washington, D.C., and Columbus, Ohio, have also adopted warning posters. The Center for Science in the Public Interest has published a booklet describing how a community can design and promote such legislation (see bibliography).

A novel program of public education specific to women is incorporated into the "Woman to Woman" program of the National Association of Junior Leagues, which began in 1984. When one considers the volume and sophistication of advertising and promotion of alcoholic beverages as symbols of sex, success, and enjoyment (particularly ads aimed at females), there's clearly a need for accurate information about the effects of alcohol on women. Public-service announcements, pamphlets, posters, and specific campaigns for campus and corporate women are sponsored by Junior Leagues at the local level as part of "Woman to Woman." Also included in the program are surveys of local intervention and treatment resources for women, an activity that often leads to improvement of women's access to care.

On the federal level, Congress has required that 5% of the funds allotted annually to the States for prevention and treatment services in the Alcohol and Drug Block Grant be devoted to new and/or expanded programs for women. This so-called "women's setaside," first required in 1984, has funded hundreds of new programs.

Other prevention efforts aimed at women involve the inclusion of education on alcohol/drugs in programs for abused women, women undergoing life transitions, pregnant women, and daughters of alcoholic parents.

Environment-oriented prevention efforts strive to counter the social pressures that encourage women to drink like men, to smoke, or to use other drugs. As American society continues to deny women social and economic equality, all measures that truly improve the status of women will also support both prevention and rehabilitation efforts.

CONCLUSION

This booklet has summarized some of the recently acquired knowledge about alcohol/drug problems in women and how to identify, diagnose, and treat them. Although increasing interest in these problems has been shown in the past decade, there are still critical gaps in knowledge about the physiological, psychological, and social aspects of these problems, including their prevention and treatment. Only through a significant investment in research and programming, and through support of beneficial public policies, will we begin to find solutions. Yet successful prevention and rehabilitation are absolutely essential for the health of present and future generations of Americans. It's up to all of us to reduce stigma, support enlightened public policies, and ensure adequate funding for prevention, treatment, and research.

APPENDIX 1:
DIAGNOSTIC QUESTIONNAIRE

1. When you are depressed or nervous, do you find that any of the following help you feel better or more relaxed?

	Very Helpful	Not Helpful	Never Tried
a. Smoking cigarettes	___	___	___
b. Working harder than usual at home or job	___	___	___
c. Taking a tranquilizer	___	___	___
d. Taking some other kind of drug or medication	___	___	___
e. Having a drink	___	___	___
f. Talking it over with friends or relatives	___	___	___

2. Think of the times you have been most depressed. At those times did you:

	Yes	No
a. Lose or gain weight?	___	___
b. Lose interest in things that usually interest you?	___	___
c. Have spells when you could not stop crying?	___	___
d. Suffer from insomnia?	___	___

3. Have you ever gone to a doctor, psychologist, social worker, counselor, or clergyman for help with an emotional problem?   ___ ___

4. How many cigarettes a day do you smoke?

   ___ more than 2 packs   ___ 1-2 packs
   ___ less than 1 pack   ___ none

5. How often do you have a drink of wine, beer, or a beverage containing alcohol?

_____ three or more times a day   _____ once or twice a week

_____ twice a day   _____ once or twice a month

_____ once almost every day   _____ less than once a month

                                            _____ never

6. a. If you drink wine, beer, or other beverages containing alcohol, how often do you have four or more drinks?

_____ almost always   _____ frequently

_____ sometimes   _____ never

   b. If you drink wine, beer, or other beverages containing alcohol, how often do you have only one or two?

_____ almost always   _____ frequently

_____ sometimes   _____ never

	Yes	No
7. Does your drinking sometimes lead to problems between you and your family, that is, wife, husband, children, parent, or close relative?	_____	_____
8. During the past year, have close relatives or friends worried or complained about your drinking?	_____	_____
9. Has a friend or family member ever told you about things you said or did while you were drinking that you do not remember?	_____	_____
10. Have you, within the past year, started to drink alcohol and found it difficult to stop before becoming intoxicated?	_____	_____
11. Has your father or mother ever had problems with alcohol?	_____	_____

APPENDIX 2:
USE OF THE QUESTIONNAIRE

The questionnaire is designed to be filled out by the patient in the waiting room. Alternatively it may be administered by a staff member. Its purpose is to alert the physician to possible alcohol problems and to the extent of self-reported smoking and alcohol use. It may alert the physician to the presence of emotional problems.

Q.1   An answer of "very helpful" on c, d, or e should alert the physician to possible alcohol/drug dependence.

Q.2-3   Any "yes" should alert the physician to possible emotional problems.

Q.7-11 Any "yes" should alert the physician to possible alcohol problems.

Q.4-6   These questions indicate the amount of cigarette and alcohol use. Although patients with alcohol problems may underreport their drinking, the recorded data may be of considerable help.

If the physician suspects or is sure that the patient has a drinking problem, he or she should:

1. Establish a firm diagnosis. Consult the National Council on Alcoholism's criteria for the diagnosis of alcoholism, or the American Psychiatric Association's Diagnostic and Statistical Manual (DSM III-R).

2. When consultation or referral is appropriate, consult or refer to:
    a. a physician experienced in the treatment of alcoholism;
    b. an alcoholism treatment facility;
    c. your local council on alcoholism;
    d. Alcoholics Anonymous. A.A. is listed in every telephone directory.

3. Refer family members and other concerned and interested persons close to the patient to:
   a. a physician experienced in the treatment of alcoholism;
   b. an alcoholism treatment facility;
   c. your local council on alcoholism;
   d. Al-Anon family groups, including Alateen for young family members. These groups may be contacted through telephone listings for Al-Anon or for Alcoholics Anonymous.

APPENDIX 3:
HEALTH QUESTIONNAIRE

1. When you are depressed or nervous, do you find that any of the following help you feel better or more relaxed?

	Very Helpful	Not Helpful	Never Tried
a. Smoking cigarettes	____	____	____
b. Working harder than usual at home or job	____	____	____
c. Taking a tranquilizer	____	____	____
d. Taking some other kind of drug or medication	____	____	____
e. Having a drink	____	____	____
f. Talking it over with friends or relatives	____	____	____

2. Think of the times you have been most depressed. At those times did you:

	Yes	No
a. Lose or gain weight?	____	____
b. Lose interest in things that usually interest you?	____	____
c. Have spells when you could not stop crying?	____	____
d. Suffer from insomnia?	____	____

3. Have you ever gone to a doctor, psychologist, social worker, counselor, or clergyman for help with an emotional problem?   ____ ____

4. How many cigarettes a day do you smoke?

____ more than 2 packs   ____ 1-2 packs
____ less than 1 pack   ____ none

5. How often do you have a drink of wine, beer, or a beverage containing alcohol?

_____ three or more times a day   _____ once or twice a week

_____ twice a day   _____ once or twice a month

_____ once almost every day   _____ less than once a month

_____ never

6. a. If you drink wine, beer, or other beverages containing alcohol, how often do you have four or more drinks?

_____ almost always   _____ frequently

_____ sometimes   _____ never

   b. If you drink wine, beer, or other beverages containing alcohol, how often do you have only one or two?

_____ almost always   _____ frequently

_____ sometimes   _____ never

7. What prescribed medications do you take? _____

_____

8. What other drugs or medications do you use? _____

_____

	Yes	No
9. Does your drinking or taking other drugs sometimes lead to problems between you and your family, that is, wife, husband, children, parent, or close relative?	_____	_____
10. During the past year, have close relatives or friends worried or complained about your drinking or taking other drugs?	_____	_____
11. Has a friend or family member ever told you about things you said or did while you were drinking or using other drugs that you do not remember?	_____	_____

12. Have you, within the past year, started to drink alcohol and found it difficult to stop before becoming intoxicated? _____ _____

13. Has your father or mother ever had problems with alcohol or other drugs? _____ _____

APPENDIX 4:
USE OF THE QUESTIONNAIRE

The questionnaire is designed to be filled out by the patient in the waiting room. Alternatively it may be administered by a staff member. Its purpose is to alert the physician to possible problems with alcohol or other drugs, and to the extent of self-reported smoking, alcohol and other drug use. It may alert the physician to the presence of emotional problems.

Q.1   An answer of "very helpful" on c, d, or e should alert the physician to possible alcohol/drug dependence.

Q.2-3   Any "yes" should alert the physician to possible emotional problems.

Q.7-11   Any "yes" should alert the physician to possible alcohol/drug problems.

Q.4-6   These questions indicate the amount of cigarette and alcohol use. Although patients with alcohol problems may underreport their drinking, the recorded data may be of considerable help.

If the physician suspects or is sure that the patient has an alcohol or other drug problem, he or she should:

1. Establish a firm diagnosis. Consult the National Council on Alcoholism's criteria for the diagnosis of alcoholism or the American Psychiatric Association's Diagnostic and Statistical Manual (DSM III-R).

2. When consultation or referral is appropriate, consult or refer to:
   a. a physician experienced in the treatment of chemical dependence;
   b. an alcoholism, addiction, or chemical dependence treatment facility;
   c. your local council on alcoholism or alcohol and other drug problems;
   d. Alcoholics Anonymous, Narcotics Anonymous, or Cocaine Anonymous. Their numbers are usually listed in telephone directories.

3. Refer family members and other concerned and interested persons close to the patient to:
   a. a physician experienced in the treatment of chemical dependence;
   b. an alcoholism, addiction, or chemical dependence treatment facility;
   c. your local council on alcoholism or alcohol and other drug problems;
   d. Al-Anon family groups, including Alateen for young family members. These groups may be contacted through telephone listings for Al-Anon or Alcoholics Anonymous, or for Narcotics Anonymous.

SUGGESTED READING

General References

AMA Council on Scientific Affairs. "Fetal Effects of Maternal Alcohol Use." *Journal of the American Medical Association* 249 (1983): 2517-21. This article by an AMA body reviews knowledge about drinking and pregnancy.

Blume, S.B. "Women and Alcohol, A Review." *Journal of the American Medical Association* 256 (Sept. 19, 1986): 1467-70. This review, with 51 references, concentrates on medical aspects of the subject.

Corrigan, E.M. *Alcoholic Women in Treatment*. New York: Oxford University Press, 1980. This book presents a study in depth of women in treatment.

Gomberg, E.L. "Women: Alcohol and Other Drugs" in B. Segal, ed., *Perspectives on Drug Use in the United States*. New York: Haworth Press, 1986. This chapter presents a broad historic and cultural view of the subject.

Greenblatt, M., and M. Schuckit, eds. *Alcoholism Problems in Women and Children*. New York: Grune & Stratton, 1976. This volume includes a review of the Jones and Jones work on blood alcohol levels in women.

Kalant, O.J., ed. *Alcohol and Drug Problems in Women*. New York: Plenum Press, 1980. This volume looks at both alcohol and other drug use.

Ray, B.A., and M.C. Braude, eds. *Women and Drugs: A New Era for Research*. Washington, D.C.: Department of Health & Human Services, NIDA Research Monograph 65, 1986.

Wilsnack, S.C., and L.S. Beckman, eds. *Alcohol Problems in Women*. New York: Plenum Press, 1980. This is an important overall reference on women and alcohol.

Women and Alcohol: Health-Related Issues. Washington, D.C.: U.S. Department of Health and Human Services, Research Monograph 16, Publication No. (ADM) 86-1139. This volume is the collected proceedings of a 1984 conference reviewing recent research findings and questions related to women and alcohol. The Wilsnack study is discussed along with other important new knowledge.

Specific References

Drugs and Pregnancy. Rockville, Maryland: American Council for Drug Education, 1986.

Beckman, L.J. "Sex-role Conflict in Alcoholic Women: Myth or Reality." *Journal of Abnormal Psychology* 84 (1978): 408-17.

Bingol, N. "The Influence of Socioeconomic Factors on the Occurrence of FAS." *Advances in Alcoholism and Substance Abuse* 6, No. 4 (1987): 105-18.

Blume, S.B. *Drinking and Pregnancy*. Minneapolis: Johnson Institute, 1981. This booklet reproduces the Women's Health Questionnaire.

Cadoret, R.J., et al. "An Adoption Study of Genetic and Environmental Factors in Drug Abuse." *Archives of General Psychiatry* 43 (1986): 1131-36.

Cermak, T.L. *Diagnosing and Treating Co-dependence*. Minneapolis: Johnson Institute, 1986.

Cloninger, C.R. "Neurogenetic Adaptive Mechanism in Alcoholism." *Science* 236 (1987): 410-16. This paper includes a summary of the Stockholm adoption study findings and proposes an integrated model of alcoholism.

Fillmore, K.M. "The Social Victims of Drinking." *British Journal of Addictions* 80 (1985): 307-14.

Fillmore, K.M., et al. *The 27 Year Longitudinal Panel Study of Drinking by Students in College*. National Institute of Alcohol Abuse and Alcoholism, 1975.

George, W.H., et al. "Male Perceptions of The Drinking Woman: Is Liquor Quicker?" Presented at Eastern Psychological Association, New York City, April 1986.

Halliday, A., et al. "Alcohol Abuse in Women Seeking Gynecologic Care." *Obstetrics and Gynecology* 68 (1986): 322-26.

Hoffman, N.G., and P.A. Harrison. *CATOR 1987 Report, Findings Two Years After Treatment*. Cator, Minn., 1986. Also available is a 1987 report on adolescent residential treatment follow-up.

Hollstedt, C., and L. Dahlgren. "Peripheral Markers in the Female 'Hidden Alcoholic.'" *Acta Psychiatrica Scandinavica* 75 (1987): 591-96.

Jones, M.C. "Personality Antecedents and Correlates of Drinking Patterns in Women." *Journal of Consultation and Clinical Psychology* 36 (1971): 61-69.

Rosett, H.L. "Reduction of Alcohol Consumption During Pregnancy with Benefits to the Newborn." *Alcoholism: Clinical and Experimental Research* 4 (1980): 178-84.

Rounsaville, B.J., et al. "Psychopathology as a Predictor of Treatment Outcome." *Alcoholics Archives of General Psychiatry*, 44 (1987): 505-13.

Schechter, D.M. *Alcohol Warning Signs: How to Get Legislation Passed in Your City*. Washington, D.C.: Center for Science in the Public Interest, 1985.

Smith, E.M., et al. "Predictors of Mortality in Alcoholic Women." *Alcoholism: Chemical and Experimental Research* 7 (1983): 237-43.

Weiner, L. "Clinical Prevention of Fetal Alcohol Effects: A Reality." *Alcohol Health & Research World* (Summer 1987), pp. 60-94.

Wilson, G.T., and D.M. Lawson. "Effects of Alcohol on Sexual Arousal in Women." *Journal of Abnormal Psychology* 85 (1976): 489-97.

Books by and about Recovering Women

Allen, C. *I'm Black and I'm Sober*. Minneapolis: CompCare, 1978.

Ford, B. *Betty: A Glad Awakening*. Garden City, New York: Doubleday, 1987.

McCambridge, M. *The Quality of Mercy*. New York: New York Times Books, 1981.

Meryman, R. *Broken Promises, Mended Dreams*. Boston: Little Brown, 1984.

Moran, M. *Lost Years*. Garden City, New York: Doubleday, 1985.

Rachel, V. *A Woman Like You*. San Francisco: Harper and Row, 1985.

Roth, L. *I'll Cry Tomorrow*. New York: Frederick Fell, 1954.

Southerby, N., and A. Southerby. *Twelve Young Women*. Long Beach, Calif.: Southerby and Associates, 1975.